COLON CANCER SURGERY RECOVERY COOKBOOK

A Comprehensive Guide To Post-Colon Cancer Surgery Recovery With Nutrient-Packed Dishes, Meal Plans, And Tips For Restoring Health And Vitality

STEPHANIE LOUDER

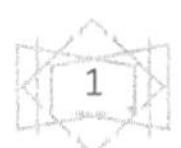

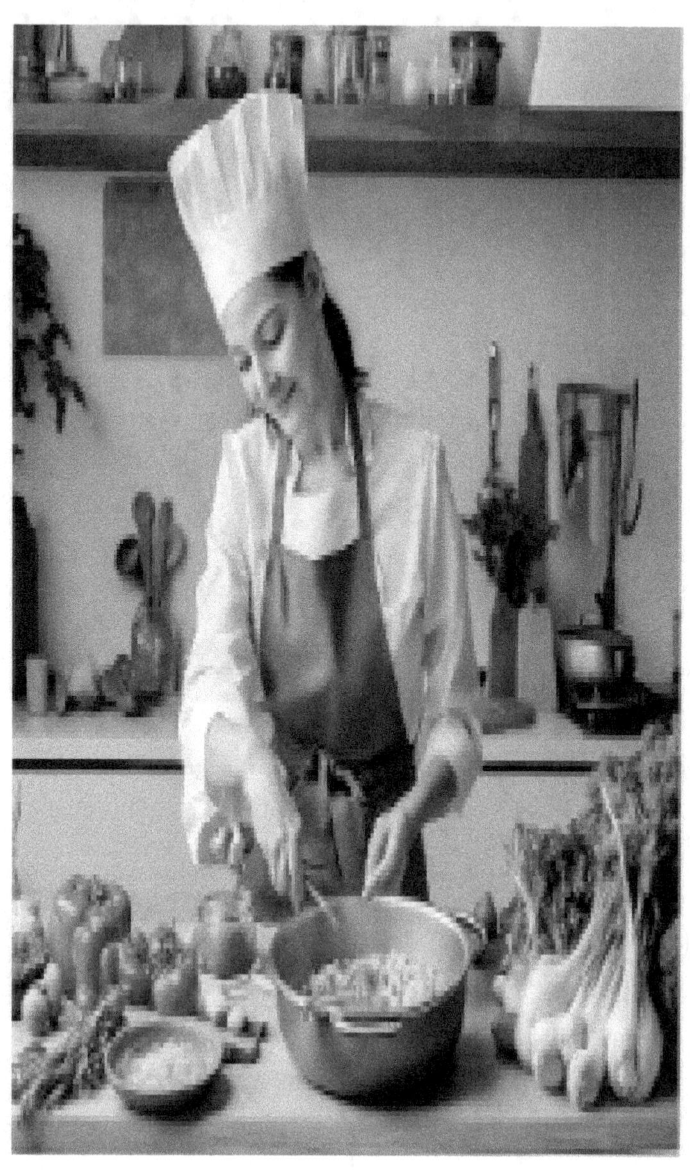

Contents

CHAPTER 1 5

Understanding Colon Cancer Surgery And Nutrition 6

Introduction to Colon Cancer Surgery Recovery: 6

Importance of Nutrition in Colon Cancer Recovery: 7

Key Nutrients for Colon Cancer Patients: 9

Foods to Include and Avoid: 10

CHAPTER 2 14

Breakfasts For Colon Cancer Surgery Recovery 14

Nutrient-Packed Breakfast Bowls 14

Energizing Smoothies and Juices 18

CHAPTER 3 21

Wholesome Main Dishes 21

CHAPTER 4 25

Brain-Boosting Meals 25

CHAPTER 5 30

Hydration And Beverages 30

CHAPTER 6 37

Snacks, Appetizers, And Desserts 37

Nutritious Snack Ideas: 37

Healthy Desserts for Treats: 40

CHAPTER 7 43

Meal Plans And Cooking Tips...........................43

Weekly Meal Plans for Different Dietary Needs
....43

Meal Prep Strategies for Convenience 45

Customizing Meal Plans for Individual Patients
....46

Conclusion 49

Copyright © 2024 Stephanie Louder.

All rights reserved.

Unauthorized reproduction or distribution of this material is prohibited. For permissions, contact Stephanie Louder at stephanielouder13@gmail.com

Disclaimer

This book authored by Stephanie Louder, is provided for informational purposes only.

Neither the author nor the publisher assumes any responsibility for the use or misuse of the information herein. This guide does not endorse or support any specific platform or method. Readers are encouraged to consult with healthcare professionals for personalized advice.

CHAPTER 1

<u>Understanding Colon Cancer Surgery And Nutrition</u>

Colon cancer surgery is a critical component of treating this disease, and proper nutrition plays a significant role in the recovery process. This section delves into the intricacies of colon cancer surgery, the importance of nutrition during recovery, key nutrients essential for colon cancer patients, and foods that should be included or avoided to support healing and overall health.

Introduction to Colon Cancer Surgery Recovery:

Colon cancer surgery is a common treatment option for patients with localized colon cancer or as part of a broader treatment plan for more advanced stages. The goal of surgery is to remove the cancerous tumor along with surrounding tissue to prevent the spread of cancer cells. Depending on the stage and location of the cancer, different surgical approaches may be used, such as segmental resection, partial colectomy, or total colectomy.

After surgery, the recovery process is crucial for patients to regain strength, heal from the procedure, and minimize the risk of complications. Recovery times can vary based on the type of surgery, overall health of the patient, and any additional treatments like chemotherapy or radiation therapy. Nutrition plays a vital role in supporting the body during this recovery phase, providing essential nutrients for healing, maintaining energy levels, and supporting overall well-being.

Importance of Nutrition in Colon Cancer Recovery:
Nutrition plays a crucial role in the recovery and overall health of colon cancer patients. Proper nutrition can help:

1.   Support Healing: Adequate nutrition is essential for the body to heal effectively after surgery. Nutrients like protein, vitamins, and minerals play key roles in tissue repair, immune function, and overall recovery.

2.	Maintain Energy Levels: Surgery and cancer treatments can often lead to fatigue and reduced energy levels. A well-balanced diet can help provide the energy needed for daily activities and promote a faster recovery.

3.	Boost Immune Function: A healthy diet rich in vitamins, antioxidants, and immune-boosting nutrients can strengthen the immune system, helping the body fight off infections and recover more efficiently.

4.	Prevent Nutrient Deficiencies: Surgery and cancer treatments can sometimes impact nutrient absorption or increase nutrient needs. By focusing on nutrient-dense foods, patients can reduce the risk of nutrient deficiencies and support optimal health.

5.	Improve Quality of Life: Eating a variety of nutritious foods can improve overall well-being, reduce side effects of treatment, and enhance quality of life during recovery.

Colon cancer patients can benefit from a well-rounded diet that includes a variety of nutrients essential for healing and overall health. Some key nutrients to focus on include:

1.   Protein: Protein is crucial for tissue repair and muscle maintenance. Good sources of protein include lean meats, poultry, fish, eggs, legumes, and dairy products.

2.   Fiber: Fiber plays a role in digestive health and can help prevent constipation, a common issue after surgery. High-fiber foods include whole grains, fruits, vegetables, and legumes.

3.   Vitamins and Minerals: Adequate intake of vitamins and minerals is important for immune function, energy production, and overall health. Focus on consuming a variety of fruits, vegetables, whole grains, and lean proteins to obtain essential vitamins like vitamin C, vitamin D, vitamin E, and minerals such as calcium, magnesium, and zinc.

4.   Omega-3 Fatty Acids: Omega-3 fatty acids have anti-inflammatory properties and may benefit colon cancer patients.

Sources of omega-3s include fatty fish (salmon, sardines), flaxseeds, chia seeds, walnuts, and soybeans.

5.   Fluids: Staying hydrated is crucial, especially after surgery. Aim to drink plenty of water throughout the day and include hydrating foods like fruits and vegetables in your diet.

Foods to Include and Avoid:

In addition to focusing on key nutrients, there are specific foods that colon cancer patients should include or avoid during recovery:

Foods to Include:

1.   Fruits and Vegetables: Colorful fruits and vegetables are rich in vitamins, minerals, antioxidants, and fiber. Aim to include a variety of produce in your diet to obtain a range of nutrients.

2.   Whole Grains: Whole grains like brown rice, quinoa, whole wheat bread, and oats provide fiber, vitamins, and minerals.

Choose whole grains over refined grains for added nutritional benefits.

3.   Lean Proteins: Opt for lean protein sources such as chicken, turkey, fish, tofu, legumes, and low-fat dairy products. These foods are rich in protein without excessive saturated fats.

4.   Healthy Fats: Include sources of healthy fats in your diet, such as avocados, nuts, seeds, and olive oil. These fats are beneficial for heart health and overall well-being.

5.   Hydrating Foods: Incorporate hydrating foods like soups, smoothies, and watery fruits (cucumber, watermelon) to maintain proper hydration levels.

Foods to Avoid:

1.   Processed Meats: Limit or avoid processed meats like bacon, sausage, and deli meats, as

they are high in saturated fats and sodium, which may not be beneficial for overall health.

2.   Sugary Foods and Drinks: Minimize intake of sugary snacks, desserts, and beverages, as they can contribute to weight gain and may not provide nutritional benefits.

3.   High-Fat Foods: While some fats are healthy, excessive intake of high-fat foods like fried foods, fatty cuts of meat, and full-fat dairy products should be limited.

4.   Alcohol: Limit alcohol consumption, as it can interfere with healing and may not be suitable for individuals undergoing cancer treatment.

5.   Caffeine: While moderate caffeine intake is generally fine, excessive caffeine consumption should be avoided, especially if it leads to dehydration or digestive issues.

By focusing on a well-balanced diet rich in essential nutrients, hydrating foods, and healthy choices, colon cancer patients can support their recovery, enhance overall health, and improve their quality of life during and after treatment. Working with a healthcare team, including a registered dietitian, can provide personalized nutrition guidance tailored to individual needs and preferences.

CHAPTER 2
Breakfasts For Colon Cancer Surgery Recovery

Nutrient-Packed Breakfast Bowls

Nutrient-packed breakfast bowls are an excellent choice for individuals recovering from colon cancer surgery. These bowls are designed to provide a balanced combination of essential nutrients that support healing and overall well-being.

One key element of nutrient-packed breakfast bowls is their versatility. They can be customized to meet specific dietary needs and preferences, making them suitable for a wide range of individuals.

In these bowls, a variety of nutrient-rich ingredients are often combined. This may include whole grains such as quinoa or oats, which provide fiber for digestive health and sustained energy. Additionally, protein sources like Greek yogurt, tofu, or nuts and seeds are commonly added to promote muscle repair and support immune function.

Fruits and vegetables play a crucial role in nutrient-packed breakfast bowls, offering vitamins, minerals, and antioxidants. Berries, bananas, spinach, and avocado are popular choices that contribute to the overall nutritional profile of the meal. Incorporating these colorful ingredients not only enhances flavor but also adds visual appeal, making the breakfast experience more enjoyable.

To further boost nutritional value, toppings such as chia seeds, flaxseeds, or hemp hearts are often included. These seeds are rich in omega-3 fatty acids, which have anti-inflammatory properties and may aid in recovery post-surgery.

Other toppings like coconut flakes, dried fruits, or granola can add texture and additional nutrients to the bowl.

Preparing nutrient-packed breakfast bowls is relatively straightforward, making them suitable for busy mornings or when energy levels may be lower during recovery.

They can be assembled ahead of time and stored in the refrigerator, allowing for quick and convenient meals.

Healing Porridges and Oatmeal Varieties

Healing porridges and oatmeal varieties are comforting and nourishing options for individuals recovering from colon cancer surgery. These warm breakfast dishes are gentle on the digestive system and can be easily customized to meet specific dietary requirements.

Oats, a key ingredient in many healing porridges and oatmeal recipes, are known for their high fiber content, which promotes healthy digestion and helps regulate blood sugar levels.

They also contain beta-glucans, a type of soluble fiber that supports immune function, making them particularly beneficial during recovery.

To enhance the healing properties of porridges and oatmeal, ingredients like ground flaxseeds, chia seeds, or nuts can be added.

These ingredients contribute healthy fats and protein, which are essential for tissue repair and overall recovery.

Incorporating fruits such as apples, berries, or dried fruits into porridges adds natural sweetness and additional vitamins and antioxidants. Spices like cinnamon or ginger not only enhance flavor but also provide anti-inflammatory benefits that can aid in post-surgery healing.

For individuals with specific dietary needs, alternative grains like quinoa or amaranth can be used to create diverse oatmeal varieties.

These grains offer unique nutritional profiles and add variety to the breakfast options, ensuring a well-rounded and satisfying meal.

Preparing healing porridges and oatmeal varieties can be done on the stovetop or in a microwave, depending on time constraints and convenience.

They can be flavored with ingredients like vanilla extract, honey, or maple syrup for added sweetness, making them appealing to different taste preferences.

Energizing smoothies and juices are refreshing options that can provide a nutrient boost for individuals recovering from colon cancer surgery. These beverages are easy to digest, making them ideal for those experiencing appetite changes or digestive discomfort post-surgery.

One of the key benefits of energizing smoothies and juices is their ability to pack a variety of nutrients into a single serving. Ingredients such as leafy greens like spinach or kale, fruits like bananas or mangoes, and protein sources like yogurt or plant-based protein powders can all be blended together to create a nutrient-dense beverage.

Leafy greens are rich in vitamins A, C, and K, as well as minerals like potassium and magnesium, which are important for overall health and recovery.

Fruits contribute natural sugars, vitamins, and antioxidants, while protein sources support muscle repair and immune function.

To enhance the energizing properties of these beverages, ingredients like ginger, turmeric, or green tea can be added.

These ingredients have anti-inflammatory and antioxidant properties, which can support the body's healing processes and boost energy levels.

For individuals with specific dietary restrictions or preferences, smoothies and juices can be customized accordingly.

Options like dairy-free smoothies using almond or coconut milk, or vegetable-based juices, provide alternatives that are still nutrient-rich and flavorful.

Preparing energizing smoothies and juices is simple and can be done using a blender or juicer.

They can be consumed as standalone breakfast options or paired with other foods for a more substantial meal. Incorporating these beverages into a post-surgery recovery diet can help ensure adequate hydration and nutrient intake, supporting overall healing and well-being.

CHAPTER 3
Wholesome Main Dishes

Wholesome Main Dishes play a crucial role in supporting overall health and recovery, especially for individuals focusing on healing and well-being. Within this category, there are several key concepts that are vital to understand and incorporate into meal planning. These concepts revolve around lean protein options for recovery, healing grains and legumes, and vegetable-centric main courses. Each of these elements contributes significantly to a balanced and nutritious diet, providing essential nutrients and promoting optimal health outcomes.

Lean protein options are essential components of wholesome main dishes, particularly for individuals recovering from illness or injury. Lean proteins are low in fat and calories but rich in essential amino acids, making them ideal for supporting muscle repair and growth, immune function, and overall recovery.

Examples of lean protein sources include poultry, such as chicken and turkey breast, fish like salmon and tuna, lean cuts of beef or pork, tofu, tempeh, legumes such as lentils and beans, and low-fat dairy products like yogurt and cottage cheese. Incorporating these protein options into main dishes ensures a well-rounded and nutrient-dense meal that supports recovery and overall health.

Healing grains and legumes are another integral part of wholesome main dishes, offering a range of health benefits and nutrients. Whole grains such as quinoa, brown rice, barley, and oats are rich in fiber, vitamins, minerals, and antioxidants.

They provide sustained energy, support digestive health, and help regulate blood sugar levels, making them valuable additions to recovery-focused meals. Legumes, including beans, lentils, and chickpeas, are also nutrient powerhouses, packed with protein, fiber, iron, and other essential nutrients. They promote satiety, aid in weight management, and contribute to heart health, making them excellent choices for wholesome main dishes.

 Combining healing grains and legumes in main courses adds depth, texture, and nutritional value to meals, supporting overall well-being and recovery.

Vegetable-centric main courses are characterized by their focus on vegetables as the central component of the dish. Vegetables are nutrient-dense foods that are rich in vitamins, minerals, antioxidants, and fiber, making them essential for overall health and recovery.

Including a variety of colorful vegetables such as leafy greens, cruciferous vegetables, bell peppers, carrots, tomatoes, and squash in main dishes adds flavor, texture, and nutritional diversity. Vegetable-centric main courses can be prepared in various ways, including roasting, grilling, sautéing, or incorporating them into soups, stews, salads, and stir-fries. By making vegetables the star of the meal, these main courses provide essential nutrients, support immune function, aid in digestion, and promote overall health and healing.

In summary, wholesome main dishes are integral to supporting recovery and promoting overall well-being. Understanding and incorporating lean protein options, healing grains and legumes, and vegetable-centric main courses into meal planning can significantly enhance the nutritional quality and effectiveness of a healing-focused diet.

By prioritizing nutrient-dense ingredients and balanced meal compositions, individuals can optimize their recovery journey and improve their overall health outcomes.

CHAPTER 4
Brain-Boosting Meals

Brain-Boosting Meals are a crucial aspect of maintaining cognitive health and supporting optimal brain function. These meals encompass a variety of food types and combinations specifically chosen for their nutritional benefits and potential to enhance brainpower.

Among the array of Brain-Boosting Meals, three categories stand out for their unique contributions: Brain-Boosting Salads and Dressings, Nourishing Soups and Stews, and Memory-Enhancing Sandwiches and Wraps.

Brain-Boosting Salads and Dressings are more than just a mix of vegetables; they are a powerhouse of nutrients essential for brain health. Starting with the base, leafy greens like spinach, kale, and arugula provide antioxidants, vitamins, and minerals crucial for cognitive function.

These greens are often paired with brain-boosting additions such as walnuts, almonds, and seeds rich in omega-3 fatty acids, known for their role in supporting brain structure and function.

The inclusion of colorful vegetables like bell peppers, tomatoes, and carrots adds not only visual appeal but also a diverse range of antioxidants and vitamins. Incorporating fruits like berries, which are packed with antioxidants and flavonoids, further enhances the brain-boosting potential of these salads.

Dressings play a significant role in Brain-Boosting Salads, not only for flavor but also for their nutritional value. Olive oil-based dressings, rich in monounsaturated fats and polyphenols, provide anti-inflammatory benefits and support cardiovascular health, indirectly benefiting brain function. Adding herbs like basil, oregano, and rosemary not only enhances the taste but also contributes antioxidants and compounds with potential cognitive benefits. Citrus-based dressings with lemon or orange juice can add a refreshing tanginess while providing vitamin C, essential for protecting brain cells from oxidative stress.

Moving on to Nourishing Soups and Stews, these dishes offer a comforting and nutrient-dense way to boost brain function. A base of homemade broth, whether vegetable or bone broth, provides essential nutrients like collagen, amino acids, and minerals that support brain health and gut integrity. Including a variety of vegetables such as broccoli, cauliflower, and leafy greens adds fiber, vitamins, and antioxidants.

Legumes like lentils and beans are excellent additions, offering protein, fiber, and complex carbohydrates that provide a steady release of energy to the brain.

Herbs and spices play a crucial role in enhancing the flavor and nutritional profile of soups and stews. Turmeric, known for its anti-inflammatory properties due to curcumin, can be added to soups for both flavor and potential cognitive benefits. Garlic and onions not only add depth to the taste but also contain compounds that support brain health. Including lean proteins like chicken, turkey, or tofu adds amino acids necessary for neurotransmitter synthesis, contributing to optimal brain function.

Memory-Enhancing Sandwiches and Wraps offer a convenient and portable way to incorporate brain-boosting ingredients into meals. Starting with a whole grain bread or wrap provides complex carbohydrates that sustain energy levels and support brain function. Including lean proteins such as grilled chicken, salmon, or plant-based alternatives like hummus or tempeh adds essential amino acids needed for neurotransmitter production. Incorporating brain-boosting fats like avocado slices or spreads provides monounsaturated fats and nutrients like vitamin E, beneficial for cognitive health.

Adding leafy greens and vegetables like spinach, kale, cucumbers, and tomatoes not only adds freshness and texture but also provides vitamins, minerals, and antioxidants. Including memory-enhancing ingredients like blueberries, known for their high levels of antioxidants and potential cognitive benefits, can elevate the brain-boosting properties of these sandwiches and wraps. Using spreads or dressings made from ingredients like Greek yogurt, tahini, or avocado can add creaminess and nutritional value, such as probiotics for gut health or omega-3 fatty acids for brain function.

The combination of these Brain-Boosting Meals provides a holistic approach to supporting brain health and cognitive function. By incorporating a variety of nutrient-dense foods, antioxidants, healthy fats, lean proteins, and memory-enhancing ingredients, individuals can create meals that not only nourish the body but also support mental clarity, focus, and overall brain performance. Regularly including these Brain-Boosting Meals as part of a balanced diet can contribute to long-term brain health and well-being.

CHAPTER 5
Hydration And Beverages

Hydration plays a crucial role in maintaining overall health, particularly for individuals undergoing treatment or recovery from conditions like colon cancer. Colon cancer patients often face challenges related to hydration due to various factors, including treatment side effects and changes in dietary habits.

Therefore, understanding hydration tips tailored to their specific needs is essential for their well-being.

Colon cancer treatments, such as surgery, chemotherapy, and radiation therapy, can cause dehydration as they may lead to increased fluid loss through sweating, vomiting, diarrhea, or decreased appetite. Additionally, some medications used in cancer treatment may have diuretic effects, further contributing to fluid imbalance. Hence, ensuring adequate hydration becomes paramount in managing these challenges.

One of the fundamental hydration tips for colon cancer patients is to drink plenty of fluids throughout the day. Water is the best choice as it hydrates without adding extra calories, sugar, or caffeine. Encouraging patients to carry a water bottle with them and setting reminders to drink regularly can help maintain hydration levels. Infusing water with natural flavors like cucumber, lemon, or mint can make it more appealing and enjoyable to drink, increasing overall fluid intake.

Monitoring urine color can also serve as a simple indicator of hydration status. Light-colored urine typically indicates good hydration, while dark-colored urine may signal dehydration. Patients should aim for pale yellow to clear urine as a sign of adequate hydration. However, it's essential to note that certain medications or supplements may affect urine color, so consulting healthcare providers for personalized advice is advisable.

Incorporating hydrating foods into the diet is another effective strategy. Fruits and vegetables with high water content, such as watermelon, cucumbers, oranges, and lettuce, not only provide hydration but also essential vitamins, minerals, and antioxidants beneficial for overall health. Including soups, broths, and smoothies made with water-rich ingredients can also contribute to hydration while offering nourishment.

Avoiding or limiting diuretic beverages like caffeinated drinks and alcohol is crucial as they can lead to increased urine output, potentially exacerbating dehydration. Instead, opting for decaffeinated beverages or herbal teas can provide hydration without the diuretic effects. However, moderation is key, and consulting healthcare professionals regarding specific dietary restrictions or recommendations is advisable.

In cases where colon cancer patients experience symptoms like diarrhea or vomiting, rehydration solutions or electrolyte-rich beverages may be recommended to replenish lost fluids and minerals. These solutions help restore electrolyte balance, which is essential for proper bodily functions, including nerve and muscle function.

Furthermore, staying hydrated can support digestive health, especially during and after colon cancer treatment. A well-hydrated body aids in maintaining regular bowel movements, preventing constipation, which is a common concern for cancer patients due to various factors like medication side effects, reduced physical activity, or dietary changes. Consuming fiber-rich foods along with adequate fluids can promote healthy digestion and bowel function.

Overall, hydration tips tailored to colon cancer patients should focus on regular fluid intake, monitoring hydration status, incorporating hydrating foods, avoiding diuretic beverages, and seeking medical advice for specific hydration needs. By prioritizing hydration, patients can better manage treatment related challenges and support their overall well-being during the recovery process.

Brain-Enhancing Drink Recipes are designed to provide not only hydration but also nutrients that support cognitive function and brain health. These recipes are especially beneficial for individuals looking to boost their mental performance or support brain health during recovery from illnesses like colon cancer. Incorporating ingredients known for their cognitive benefits, these drinks offer a refreshing and nutritious way to nourish the brain.

One of the key ingredients often included in brain-enhancing drink recipes is green tea. Green tea contains catechins and antioxidants that have been linked to improved cognitive function, memory, and focus. Brewing green tea and incorporating it into smoothies or iced teas with added fruits like berries, which are rich in antioxidants and vitamins, creates a refreshing brain-boosting beverage.

Another popular ingredient in brain-enhancing drinks is blueberries. Blueberries are known for their high levels of antioxidants, particularly flavonoids like anthocyanins, which have been associated with better brain health and cognitive performance. Blending blueberries with yogurt, almond milk, or coconut water creates a delicious and nutrient-packed smoothie that supports brain function.

Omega-3 fatty acids are essential nutrients for brain health, and incorporating sources like flaxseeds, chia seeds, or walnuts into drink recipes adds a dose of these beneficial fats.

Omega-3s have been linked to improved mood, memory, and cognitive abilities, making them valuable additions to brain-enhancing beverages.

Turmeric, a spice known for its anti-inflammatory and antioxidant properties, is often included in brain-enhancing drink recipes. Turmeric contains curcumin, which has been studied for its potential cognitive benefits, including protection against neurodegenerative diseases. Combining turmeric with ginger, lemon, and honey in a warm tea or golden milk latte creates a soothing and brain-boosting drink option.

Incorporating leafy greens like spinach or kale into smoothies or green juices adds vitamins, minerals, and phytonutrients that support brain health. These greens are rich in folate, vitamin K, and antioxidants, contributing to overall cognitive function and neuroprotection.

Herbal teas infused with ingredients like ginkgo biloba, gotu kola, or rosemary are also popular choices for brain-enhancing drinks. These herbs have been traditionally used for their cognitive-enhancing properties and can be enjoyed as hot or cold beverages, depending on preference.

Hydration is a fundamental aspect of brain health, and these brain-enhancing drink recipes not only provide essential fluids but also deliver nutrients that support cognitive function, memory, and overall brain wellness. Incorporating a variety of brain-boosting ingredients into daily hydration routines can contribute to mental clarity, focus, and long-term brain health benefits.

CHAPTER 6
Snacks, Appetizers, And Desserts

Creating a well-rounded recovery-focused cookbook involves careful consideration of snacks, appetizers, and desserts. These elements play a crucial role in the overall nutritional balance of a meal plan, providing not just sustenance but also enjoyment and satisfaction. Let's delve deeper into each of these categories to understand how they can be optimized for recovery.

Nutritious Snack Ideas:

Snacks are often seen as quick bites to curb hunger between meals, but in a recovery-focused context, they serve a more significant purpose. Nutritious snacks should not only provide energy but also deliver essential nutrients that support the body's healing processes. Here are some ideas for nutritious snacks:

1. Trail Mix Varieties: Create custom trail mixes using nuts, seeds, dried fruits, and perhaps

some dark chocolate for a satisfying blend of protein, healthy fats, and antioxidants.

2.   Greek Yogurt Parfaits: Layer Greek yogurt with fresh fruits, granola, and a drizzle of honey for a snack rich in probiotics, calcium, and fiber.

3.   Homemade Energy Bars: Make energy bars using oats, nuts, seeds, and dried fruits bound together with natural sweeteners like honey or dates. These bars can be customized to include ingredients like chia seeds or protein powder for added nutrition.

4.   Vegetable Sticks with Hummus: Pair colorful vegetable sticks like carrots, cucumbers, and bell peppers with homemade hummus for a snack packed with vitamins, minerals, and healthy fats.

5.   Smoothie Bowls: Blend together fruits, leafy greens, Greek yogurt or plant-based protein, and a liquid like almond milk to create a nutrient-dense smoothie bowl topped with seeds, nuts, and fresh fruit slices.

These snack ideas not only offer nutritional benefits but also cater to different taste preferences and dietary restrictions, making them versatile additions to a recovery meal plan.

Appetizers for Recovery:

Appetizers set the tone for a meal, offering a preview of flavors and textures while stimulating the appetite. In a recovery-focused cookbook, appetizers can be designed to complement the main dishes while providing additional nutritional value. Here are some appetizer ideas suitable for recovery:

1.	Grilled Vegetable Skewers: Marinate colorful vegetables like bell peppers, zucchini, and mushrooms in herbs and olive oil before grilling for a flavorful appetizer rich in antioxidants and fiber.

2.	Quinoa-Stuffed Bell Peppers: Stuff bell peppers with a quinoa and vegetable mix seasoned with herbs and spices for a protein-packed appetizer that's also gluten-free.

3.   Smoked Salmon Rolls: Roll smoked salmon slices with cream cheese, avocado, and fresh herbs for a delicious appetizer high in omega-3 fatty acids and protein.

4.   Caprese Salad Skewers: Skewer cherry tomatoes, fresh mozzarella balls, and basil leaves drizzled with balsamic glaze for a refreshing appetizer bursting with flavor and nutrients.

5.   Cucumber Cups with Tuna Salad: Hollow out cucumber slices to create cups filled with a light tuna salad mixed with Greek yogurt, lemon juice, and herbs for a low-carb, high-protein appetizer option.

These appetizers not only tantalize the taste buds but also contribute to the overall nutritional profile of a meal, incorporating key nutrients essential for recovery.

Healthy Desserts for Treats:

Desserts are often associated with indulgence, but in a recovery-focused context, they can be transformed into nutrient-rich treats that satisfy cravings while supporting healing and well-being. Here are some ideas for healthy desserts:

1. Fruit and Yogurt Parfaits: Layer fresh fruits like berries, kiwi, and mango with Greek yogurt and a sprinkle of granola or nuts for a satisfying dessert packed with vitamins, minerals, and probiotics.

2. Chia Seed Pudding: Make chia seed pudding using almond milk or coconut milk, sweetened with a touch of honey or maple syrup, and topped with fresh fruit or nuts for a fiber-rich, omega-3 boosted dessert.

3. Baked Apples with Cinnamon: Core apples and bake them with a sprinkle of cinnamon and a drizzle of honey until tender for a comforting dessert that's high in fiber and antioxidants.

4. Dark Chocolate Avocado Mousse: Blend ripe avocados with cocoa powder, a natural sweetener like agave or dates, and a hint of vanilla extract for a creamy, decadent mousse rich in healthy fats and antioxidants.

5.   Frozen Yogurt Bark: Spread Greek yogurt onto a baking sheet, top with fruits, nuts, and a drizzle of honey, then freeze until firm before breaking into pieces for a refreshing, customizable dessert option.

These healthy dessert ideas showcase that indulgence can align with nutritional goals, offering sweetness without compromising on health benefits. Incorporating such desserts into a recovery-focused meal plan adds variety and enjoyment while supporting overall well-being.

In conclusion, snacks, appetizers, and desserts in a recovery-focused cookbook play pivotal roles in providing essential nutrients, stimulating appetite, and offering satisfying culinary experiences. By crafting nutritious snack options, appetizers that complement main meals, and healthy desserts, the cookbook can cater to diverse tastes and dietary needs while promoting holistic recovery and well-being.

CHAPTER 7
Meal Plans And Cooking Tips

Creating effective meal plans is a crucial aspect of nutrition, especially for individuals with specific dietary needs or health concerns. Whether it's managing weight, addressing nutritional deficiencies, or catering to medical conditions, well-designed meal plans can make a significant difference in overall health and well-being.

In this discussion, we'll delve into the concepts of weekly meal plans for different dietary needs, meal prep strategies for convenience, and customizing meal plans for individual patients.

Weekly Meal Plans for Different Dietary Needs

Designing weekly meal plans involves considering various dietary needs, preferences, and health goals. For individuals following specific diets like vegetarian, vegan, ketogenic, or gluten-free, the meal plan must be tailored to ensure they meet their nutritional requirements while enjoying a variety of flavors and textures.

It's essential to include a balance of macronutrients (carbohydrates, proteins, and fats) and micronutrients (vitamins and minerals) in each meal to support overall health.

For example, a vegetarian meal plan may include a variety of plant-based protein sources such as legumes, tofu, tempeh, and nuts, along with plenty of fruits, vegetables, whole grains, and healthy fats like avocado and olive oil. On the other hand, a ketogenic meal plan focuses on high-fat, moderate-protein, and low-carbohydrate foods such as fatty fish, eggs, avocados, nuts, seeds, and non-starchy vegetables.

When designing meal plans, it's crucial to consider individual calorie needs, activity levels, and any specific dietary restrictions or food allergies. Consulting with a registered dietitian or nutritionist can be beneficial in creating personalized meal plans that are nutritionally balanced and aligned with individual goals.

Meal preparation is key to maintaining healthy eating habits, especially for busy individuals or families. Effective meal prep strategies can save time, reduce stress, and ensure that nutritious meals are readily available throughout the week. Here are some meal prep tips for convenience:

1.   Batch Cooking: Prepare larger quantities of food items such as grains, proteins, and vegetables and store them in portion-sized containers for quick and easy meals during the week.

2.   Pre-cut and Washed Produce: Wash, chop, and store fruits and vegetables ahead of time to streamline meal preparation. This makes it easier to add fresh produce to meals without the hassle of chopping and cleaning each time.

3.   Use Slow Cookers or Instant Pots: Slow cookers and Instant Pots are great tools for preparing soups, stews, and one-pot meals with minimal effort. Simply add ingredients, set the timer, and enjoy a delicious meal later.

4.   Freeze Meals: Prepare and freeze meals in advance, such as casseroles, lasagnas, or soups, for quick reheating on busy days. Labeling and dating frozen meals can help with organization and meal planning.

5.   Pre-portion Snacks: Portion out snacks like nuts, seeds, dried fruits, or yogurt into grab-and-go containers or bags to have healthy snacks readily available when hunger strikes.

6.   Create a Meal Prep Schedule: Set aside dedicated time each week for meal prep, such as Sundays or weekends, to plan meals, grocery shop, and prepare ingredients for the upcoming week.

Customizing Meal Plans for Individual Patients

Customizing meal plans for individual patients involves a comprehensive assessment of their nutritional needs, health goals, medical conditions, food preferences, and lifestyle factors. Here are key considerations when customizing meal plans:

1.   Medical Conditions: For patients with specific medical conditions such as diabetes, hypertension, or gastrointestinal disorders, meal plans must align with dietary guidelines recommended by healthcare professionals. This may involve monitoring carbohydrate intake, sodium levels, fiber intake, or avoiding certain food triggers.

2.   Nutritional Requirements: Assessing individual calorie needs, macronutrient distribution (carbohydrates, proteins, fats), and micronutrient intake (vitamins, minerals) is essential in creating balanced meal plans that support overall health and well-being.

3.   Food Preferences: Take into account patients' food preferences, cultural background, and culinary traditions when designing meal plans. Incorporating familiar foods and flavors can enhance adherence to the meal plan and promote enjoyment of meals.

4. Lifestyle Factors: Consider patients' lifestyle factors such as work schedule, physical activity level, meal timing preferences, and cooking skills when customizing meal plans. Providing practical and achievable recommendations ensures that meal plans fit seamlessly into their daily routine.

5. Allergies and Intolerances: Identify and accommodate any food allergies, intolerances, or sensitivities when creating meal plans. Offer alternative food options and substitutions to ensure safety and prevent adverse reactions.

6. Monitoring and Adjustments: Regularly monitor patients' progress, dietary adherence, and nutritional status. Adjust meal plans as needed based on feedback, changes in health status, or evolving dietary goals.

By customizing meal plans to meet individual patients' needs, preferences, and health goals, healthcare professionals can empower patients to make positive dietary choices and improve their overall health and well-being.

Collaboration between patients, healthcare providers, and nutrition experts is essential in developing effective and sustainable meal plans that support long-term success.

Conclusion

the Colon Cancer surgery recovery cookbook provides a comprehensive guide to understanding the role of nutrition in post-surgery recovery.

It emphasizes the importance of key nutrients, offers a range of delicious recipes tailored to support healing, and provides practical tips for meal planning and preparation.

By focusing on nutrient-packed breakfasts, wholesome main dishes, brain-boosting meals, hydration strategies, and convenient snacks and desserts, this cookbook aims to help patients navigate their recovery journey with nourishing and satisfying meals. Customizable meal plans cater to different dietary needs, ensuring that each patient can find suitable options for their individual recovery needs.

www.ingramcontent.com/pod-product-compliance
Lightning Source LLC
Chambersburg PA
CBHW051708250726
48653CB00007B/2924